FreshSteps FootCare

Simple Guide to Maintaining Health Feet

APRYL M. MOORE

FresSteps FootCare
Copyright @ 2023 By Apryl M. Moore
All rights reserved

Published by FreshSteps Medical Foot and Nail Spa® LLC
McKinney, Texas

No part of this publication may be reproduced, stored, in a retrieval system, or transmitted in any form or by any means – electronic, mechanical, digital, photocopy, recording, or any other – except for brief quotations in printed reviews, without the prior permission of the publisher.

ISBN: 9798852757418

Printed in the United States of America

TABLE OF CONTENTS

Acknowledgments		v
Introduction		vii
1	Cleaning Your Feet	1
2	Infected Toenails and Skin	5
3	Thick Toenails	9
4	Calluses and Corns	12
5	Teaching Our Children Proper Foot Care	15
6	Home Care	17
7	Our Responsibility to Maintain Healthy Feet	19
8	Nail Salons Are Not Created Equally	21
9	Orthotics	24
10	Bonus Foot Care Tips	26
11	Doctor's Corner	29
Conclusion		35
Resources		37

ACKNOWLEDGMENTS

This book would not have been possible without the contribution of the key players. It is with humbleness and gratitude that I acknowledge and thank each of you.

My clients, new and old, it is because you chose me to be your service provider and trusted me with the care of your feet; you put in the work and trusted me and the process you have taught me many things, and I am grateful for the opportunity to serve you.

My daughter, Angel, now my coworker and my legacy—thank you for deciding after college you wanted to start your career alongside me, for being diligent in your education and training in foot care, for caring for our clients as I do, and for believing in this business and the services we provide to show up every day.

John Baca, DPM, FACFAS, FFPM RCPS (Glasg), thank you for trusting me enough to refer clients and understanding that what I do is only a complement to what you do. Thank you for recognizing that what we do together only benefits our clients, and they are all that matters.

INTRODUCTION

I have been an active person since I can remember, starting at a very young age at the YMCA in Chicago, IL, with swimming, gymnastics, cheerleading, ballet, and tennis. I continued swimming until the end of high school. After college, I got back into tennis and a little physical fitness, and now, I'm happy just walking and practicing yoga.

In high school, I wanted to become a surgical nurse. After doing clinicals in a nursing home to become a certified nursing assistant, I quickly realized that this may not be the career for me, and I finished with a master's degree in human resources management.

In the interim of transitioning from high school to college, I was recruited into doing nails. I absolutely loved it, but back then, doing nails was not considered a viable career choice. The goal was to graduate college and get a good job.

Today, although I am not working in the field I am qualified in, my education, business experience, and nail care experience have brought me to this point in my life, and I couldn't be happier.

The foot care I provide falls under my manicurist license for the state of Texas. I have invested in additional training to advance my skills and knowledge to be able to provide foot care for clients who would not otherwise go to a traditional nail salon due to health issues, problem toenails, or because they want a safe and private service.

Part of my advanced training required me to understand the cleaning, sanitizing, and sterilization protocols of Texas state. It required me to intern under a podiatrist. I have also taken advanced training in oncology care to understand how the different types of cancer treatments affect the body and the mental and emotional mindset of people who are currently in treatment or who have undergone treatment. All this training (advanced nail technician, certified medical nail technician, oncology-trained nail technician, and podiatrist assistant) has led me to seek out the best products on the market for foot care available to me as a nail technician, become an educator for that product line for others to better understand the product, and effectively use it on my clients.

However, it is my personal experience and the experience of working with thousands of clients to restore the health of their feet that inspired me to write this book. In this book, I share what I didn't know, what I learned, and what I have personally accomplished in foot care as a reminder to you that having a basic foot care regimen can have your feet outlast you.

Let me be clear; foot issues do not discriminate. As a young child, I remember suffering from athlete's feet. At the time, I had no idea what it was. My son, at the age of eight, suffered from the same condition due to my negligence in not giving him proper guidance on foot care.

Anyone can suffer from foot issues irrespective of age, nationality, or lifestyle.

I am Apryl Moore, Medical Nail Technician (MNT), and I am writing this book for you as a guide and a reminder that our feet are our foundation; they hold the weight we carry and carry us through life. Don't neglect them.

1

CLEANING YOUR FEET

This may seem so simple, but can we honestly say we were taught how to clean our feet? I mean really. We were taught how to wash ourselves and take a shower or bath, but for the most part, we weren't really given clear instructions on how to clean our feet or told about the importance of clean feet. I know I wasn't.

When I speak to most of my clients and we talk about how they wash their feet, most of them stop at the top and let the water do the rest. Think about it. How do you clean your feet?

Believe it or not, our feet are not as complicated as we may think.

There are only three basic things and a bonus that we need to do for our feet to keep them healthy: clean, moisturize, and clip your toenails. Everything else is just to make you feel good.

Cleaning

It is very simple and easy to clean your feet properly. Just wash them with soap and water, making sure to clean the top, sides, and bottom of your feet and in between the toes. Some people think that soaking will keep their feet healthy. Soaking just makes your feet feel good. When I talk about maintaining good health I'm talking about good foot hygiene, and soap and water in the bath or shower will do the trick.

Drying

Drying your feet after bathing/showering, swimming in the pool or sea, sweating, and so on, is very important. You don't want to skip this part when we are talking about good foot hygiene. Ignoring this step can be the cause of some very annoying problems, such as foot odor, bacteria, or fungus. Fungus and bacteria develop and thrive in moist dark places and can cause foot odor. Drying the feet completely can help prevent this.

Towel dry your feet after getting out of the bath/shower, pool, or sea. Make sure to wipe under the feet and in between the toes right away. Afterward, allow your feet to get some air for a minute or two before pulling on socks and shoes.

After returning home from work or a workout, and for kids when they come in from sports or outdoor activities, take your shoes off and wipe down your feet and change into footwear that allows your feet to air out, trying not to keep the toes covered.

Moisturize

This may take some getting used to if it is something you don't do or don't do often. Many people mistake callused skin for dry skin. I often get clients who say they have calluses when, in reality, the skin on their feet is extremely dry and in need of moisture. Many clients say, "I apply lotion on my feet, and they still feel dry." Why is that? Our feet have the thickest layer of skin on the body, and our face has the thinnest layer of skin, so just like you have an exclusive facial regimen, you also need a special foot regimen. You need a moisturizer that penetrates through all the layers of skin on the feet and stays moisturized. A lotion may penetrate the layers, but it dries out quickly, and creams may be too thick to penetrate the layers. The ideal foot moisturizer is designed primarily for the feet, and you won't need socks on to help it work.

In our salon, we use a Food and Drug Administration (FDA) cleared foam moisturizer created for foot care. It is light and designed to penetrate the layers of skin on the feet and stay in to moisturize and heal the skin.

Bonus: Disinfect

I'm all about maintaining good foot health, and as a bonus to make sure you are keeping away surface germs and bacteria, it is always good to disinfect your shoes and socks. You want to turn your socks inside out and spray them before putting them on. Find a good disinfecting spray of your choice and spray out your shoes and socks daily. This will help with bad odors and fighting surface bacteria and germs and help to prevent the spread of fungus. Also, switch up your footwear; try not to wear the same shoes every day.

Maintaining healthy feet should be a part of your daily regimen. Paying attention to your feet and touching your feet should never be considered dirty; it is a vital part of your body that needs just as much, if not more, care as any other part of your body. By doing this, you will get into the habit of looking at your feet regularly and will notice if your feet or your toenails are changing.

I understand that many people may suffer from a lack of flexibility for various reasons, may not have great vision, or may not have the proper tools or products to use. Many of my clients are unable to reach or see their feet to cut their toenails safely. If this applies to you, please seek the assistance of a family member, caretaker, or professional.

2

INFECTED TOENAILS AND SKIN

Many clients come to me by doctor's referral or in desperation to find someone who can help them with what appears to be a problem with their toenails. Some have just recently noticed that something is different with their toenails and want to find out why, some feel pain around their toenails and think it's an ingrown toenail, and some have suffered with unsightly toenails for years and just wanted to find someone who could help. Whatever the situation, clients come to me for all kinds of issues. The question I hear most often is: What is wrong with my toenails?

The truth of the matter is, for you to really know if you have a fungus or bacterial infection on your toenails or your feet, it must be tested by your primary care provider or a podiatrist. They will take a clipping of your toenails and send them to a lab to get a proper diagnosis.

Here is where the importance of checking your feet daily comes in. If you start to notice some changes in your toenails or irritation with the skin on your feet, it may be time to see your doctor. Below are some characteristics of infected toenails and skin.

Skin:
Peeling on the bottom of the feet
Peeling in between the toes
Redness
Itchiness
Excessive dryness

Toenails:
Thick
Discolored
White spots
Lifting from the nailbed
Crumbly nails
Ridges in the toenails

If you notice any kind of break in the skin or bruising on the toenails, don't wait until it gets bad. Seek professional help to identify if it is something you should be concerned about.

What causes infected skin or toenails?

There can be several causes for infected skin and toenails. Listed below are the most common ones that I've been made aware of in the years I've been servicing clients.

Trauma: Dropping something heavy on the toenail and not getting it treated, hitting the toe against a hard surface, someone stepping on the toe, ill-fitting shoes rubbing against the toenails.

Drying the feet: Not drying in between the toes, not completely drying your feet, and covering wet feet in socks and shoes are common causes of athlete's foot. It is important to remember that fungi and bacteria thrive in moist dark places. Keeping your feet covered can accelerate the problem.

Pedicures: Having pedicures in a place that has infected tools, unclean footbaths, or unclean tools, or the improper cutting of toenails.

Other people: Sharing shoes with someone who has infected feet, walking barefoot in wet places, walking barefoot in the same place as someone with infected feet, or trying on shoes at a store with no socks, where the person before could've had infected feet.

Medications: Always understand the side effects of any medications you are taking and pay attention to any changes in your body, as well as your feet, when you start taking medications. Some medications can dry out your skin, especially if you are not drinking enough water.

Compromised autoimmune system: If your immune system is compromised from any illness or you are lacking in nutrients, that, too, can cause a problem.

How to Heal Infected Skin and Toenails

When toenails and the skin on the feet become infected, for the most part, it isn't life-threatening. However, it can be annoying and embarrassing and make you feel ashamed or uncomfortable, which is why we tend to hide our feet when we start to see a problem and we don't know what to do. Most people's instinct is to cover it up.

Take action: When you see a problem starting to occur, act fast. It takes longer to cure the problem than it takes to develop the problem. Be persistent and patient during the healing process.

Seek professional help: If you see something unusual on your feet, go to a doctor and get it checked out. You can get a treatment or prescription that will start the healing process.

Find a certified medical nail tech: For example, Fresh-Steps Medical Foot and Nail Spa® can work in conjunction with your doctor or the treatment plan. We can provide you with a service that will clean your feet, clip off any unattached nails safely, reduce the thickness of a nail to allow the treatment to penetrate through, and advise you if the treatment is working or if you need to go back to the doctor.

At FreshSteps, we use FDA-cleared products that have been proven to work and are safe for our clients, along with medical-grade safe tools that keep us within the scope of our license and keep our clients safe. As medical nail techs, we have interned under a podiatrist and have been trained to recognize a potential problem to be referred to a doctor.

Doctors have a selection of medications they can prescribe, from topicals to orals, depending on the severity of the problem, which can help with the healing process of infected toenails and skin on the feet.

Healing anything first starts with identifying the problem.

3

THICK TOENAILS

This is a biggie in my salon. Many clients ask, "Why are my toenails so thick?"

Thick toenails aren't always infected. In the last chapter, we talked about infected toenails, and thick toenails can be one of the characteristics of infected toenails. But just because they are thick doesn't mean they are infected.

In my salon, I see over a hundred clients a month, and some just have thick toenails and they associate that with having a problem because their toenails weren't always like that.

Yes, it is true that over time, as we age, things change.

The thickening of toenails can happen for various reasons. I'll share the two most common reasons I've seen in my salon.

Trauma

Although we talked about how trauma can cause thick infected toenails in our previous chapter, it can also be caused without infection. It is very common when people wear ill-fitting shoes or for athletes, who are constantly moving in their shoes. Accidents, like dropping something heavy on the toenail or hitting the toenail against a hard surface can also be the causes.

In these instances, if the trauma was never addressed and continued for a long time, the toenails will not go back to their natural state; they will continue to grow out thick.

Aging

As we age, our bodies change, and one of the changes can be thicker toenails. Our bones also tend to soften and not heal as fast as they did when we were younger. This can cause our toenails to take on a different shape and possibly rub against another toe, producing friction that can cause a toenail to thicken or form a callus.

When the toenails start to thicken, it can also cause other changes, with the toenails starting to curve more than they have before, which can then cause involuted toenails. Nails that thicken and aren't cut and cleaned properly or allowed to grow too long can also become ingrown and very painful, which may lead to an infected toenail.

Another issue I see in many of my aging clients (forty plus) is pincer toenails. This is when the toenail starts to thicken and grow out to a point, and it gets worse as the toenail is allowed to grow out past the nailbed. This can be very painful and is sometimes mistaken for an ingrown toenail. Thick toenails aren't always infected toenails. However, if allowed to grow too long, and if they aren't cared for, they can become ingrown, infected, and cause a lot of pain.

Healing Thick Toenails
If your toenails have become thick due to the reasons listed above, I am sorry to say there is really no solution for it—there is no magic pill or cream that will fix it. The best option is to seek out the professional services of a licensed nail tech that specializes in foot care to keep your toenails cut, cleaned, and shaped properly, and if need be, reduce the thickness to give you comfort.

4

CALLUSES AND CORNS

Calluses and corns can be extremely irritating and painful. Often, one is mistaken for the other, so let's talk about it. We will start with the difference between the two.

Corns
Corns are generally small and deep, typically found at the top of the toe or on the side of the toe and sometimes in between. Corns have a hard layer of skin over the top, giving the appearance of a callus, but the biggest difference between a corn and a callus is that corns are generally sore to the touch. There is a very sharp pain when you touch them. Corns have a core, meaning they develop from the inside out.

Calluses
Calluses develop on the pressure points of the feet, around the heels or the balls of the feet, alongside the big toes and

the smaller toes; they can also be found on the front of the toes. Calluses form from friction or constant rubbing against the skin. They are much larger than corns, harder, and often have a yellowish tint.

Calluses develop to protect the good skin underneath. They don't generally cause pain, but if allowed to develop, they can get very hard and crack the skin. They can also become sore and create an entryway for infection. For autoimmune-compromised clients, this can be very dangerous.

What causes corn and calluses?
Corn and calluses are caused by friction—repeated rubbing against the skin. Some sources of repeated action can come from:

Ill-fitting shoes
Imbalance in the body (bad knees or hips)
Excessive weight on the feet
Not wearing socks with shoes

How do I get rid of corn and calluses?
To get rid of calluses or corns, you first must identify why you are getting them. When you do that, you solve your problem. Until then you have a few options:

Go to a podiatrist. In my salon, I don't dig out the corns, but I do use professional tools that take down the hard layers of skin without cutting, leaving the skin nice and smooth. I also have professional retail products to help soften and heal the skin. If the pain persists, I recommend my clients see a podiatrist to remove the core of the corn. They can dig out the core of your corn or have other means of getting rid of it. They can shave down calluses with a scapple.

Custom orthotics can help balance out your feet, relieving the pressure of the friction, thereby giving your feet relief and removing the issue causing the corn.

Another option is to try over-the-counter treatments.

But again, all these are temporary fixes. If you haven't identified the problem that is causing the repeated rubbing against the skin and stopped it, you won't get rid of them; they will keep coming back.

5

TEACHING OUR CHILDREN PROPER FOOT CARE

I thought this was an important chapter to include because, in my salon, I have serviced clients as young as six years old, and having dealt with my son when he had athlete's feet at the age of eight made me feel like the worst mom ever. I even have godchildren old enough to have their own children and had to clip an ingrown toenail from my six-month-old Godchild. This is just so you know that foot issues don't discriminate.

From conversations with my clients, I've discovered that many of them weren't taught proper foot care. and so they rely on Dr. Google to find out how to fix their foot issues. Dr. Google can be right about something, but sometimes, there can be too much information, and everything doesn't apply to everybody.

I always live by the motto, "Keep it simple." As mentioned earlier in this book, our feet don't require a lot.

Teaching our children some basic foot care tips can take them a long way.

Shoes: Make sure children have the correct shoes for their activities and that they are a good fit. I know kids grow fast, but too big shoes can be a problem.

Communication: Ask your child to tell you when they feel like the shoes are too tight or they start hurting their feet.

Cleaning: Show them how to clean the top and bottom of their feet and between the toes with a washcloth.

Drying: Show them how to dry their feet, top, bottom, and between the toes. When they come in after activities, tell them to take off their shoes and socks and let their feet air out.

Moisturize: Make sure they are moisturizing their feet daily with a good foot moisturizer

Clip toenails: Children's toenails tend to be thin. Don't let them rip off their toenails. If you are not comfortable with clipping their toenails, file them down or take them someplace you feel is safe and have their toenails clipped and shaped.

Check-in: Every now and then, check their feet, just in case they forget to tell you something is wrong.

Teaching your children these simple steps now can save them from growing into adults with foot issues and making bad decisions about footwear.

6

HOME CARE

In the previous chapters of this book, we have covered a few basic things about how to care for your feet and recognize toenail issues.

At FreshSteps Medical Foot and Nail Spa® LLC, when you come in with foot issues, it is my goal to educate you on what I see is going on with your feet based on my experience and knowledge, provide the best service for the issue, let you know what your return service should be, and graduate you to home care, bringing your feet back to a healthy condition so you can maintain your foot care at home. Some people, because of restrictions or because they just enjoy their service and time with me, choose to come back on a schedule for their routine foot care, and that is perfectly fine.

The objective is to make sure you understand how to maintain healthy feet, and if you must go to another service provider, that you know what to expect and how to communicate your expectations. If you choose to maintain your services at home, you must know what to do.

I want you to understand that if you come to me or any service provider, your pedicures should last at least 24–48 hours. The average time between visits for my clients is four to six weeks, depending on how fast their toenails grow. That is a lot of time between visits. In the meantime, something needs to be done, and that is where maintenance comes in—cleaning, drying, moisturizing, and possibly disinfecting.

I'll let you in on a little secret. If you are doing the maintenance between visits, you will develop the habit of touching and looking at your feet, so if something arises, you can catch it right away and act.

You will notice any new cracks in the skin, you will notice if a shoe caused a callus, you will notice if your toenail is lifting, cracked, or starting to become discolored. You will be able to identify when and how the problem started. You will be amazed at how many people tell me they have had this problem all their life, probably not but it has been a long time.

When you are doing home care, there are a few things I want you to remember:

Clean your feet daily.
Dry your feet completely.
Moisture your feet daily (twice a day is recommended) with a foot moisturizer—keep your moisturizer out where you can see it.
Keep your toenails cut low.

7

OUR RESPONSIBILITY TO MAINTAIN HEALTHY FEET

Have you ever heard the saying, "Faith without works is dead"? You cannot get the results you are expecting if you don't put in the work. I'm here to help get you through the process. It's not going to happen overnight, but you have to trust the process; sometimes it can take up to 12 months, sometimes more, sometimes less.

At FreshSteps Medical Foot and Nail Spa®, our technicians are state-licensed manicurists, advanced-licensed nail technicians, certified medical nail technicians, podiatry assistants, and oncology trained. We have gone through countless hours of training and studies to give you the highest levels of care and the safest service. We service over a thousand clients a year only in foot care. We are committed to our clients and always strive for the best results. We use FDA-cleared medical-grade products that have been tested and proven to give you the best results.

We use medical-grade tools to give you the safest service and keep up with the latest and greatest in technology and techniques. We use our proprietary waterless pedicure steps to give you the best experience.

Our responsibility is to educate and guide you through the process, as well as keep an eye out for any good or bad changes that we see during your service.

Our responsibility to you is to recognize and refer you to medical professionals if we see something out of our scope of practice. We take your care seriously.

Your responsibility is to show up for scheduled appointments every four to six weeks.

Your responsibility is to communicate any changes you have seen or felt in your feet and toenails or any discomfort or changes in your health conditions.

You need to be consistent in your treatments from us or the doctor for home care.

It's that simple. Teamwork!

This goes for any service provider you are seeing. If you are not comfortable with the level of care you are receiving from your service provider, nail technician, or doctor, seek out another professional for services.

8

NAIL SALONS ARE NOT CREATED EQUALLY

No, all nail salons or nail technicians/manicurists are not created equal! When a nail technician gets licensed, they go through basic textbook and hands-on training, and depending on what state they are in determines the number of hours they need to be in school to sit for the licensing test. Most nail technicians go to school because they want to learn how to make nails look pretty; they are in it for the art of nails.

Most advanced nail education classes are taken after the nail technicians/manicurists are licensed and have invested in additional advanced training and certifications. Other nail technicians rely on YouTube or other social media outlets to learn new techniques or skills. Ask questions of your service provider to find out if they are a good fit for you.

Truth be told, this industry is saturated with licensed and unlicensed nail technicians, and it is up to the consumer to research and choose wisely.

Find someone who specializes in the care that you need for your feet.

If their website, Google, or social media presence doesn't address your needs, move on.

Find someone you can talk to if you have special needs or any questions.

Don't be afraid to share your health issues. A seasoned professional will know the best way to care for your feet for your specific health issues.

If you are being serviced somewhere and are uncomfortable, it's okay to stop the service.

If you go in for a service and your gut is telling you something is wrong, it is. Look around and make sure it's up to the standards you are expecting. If it is not, leave.

Observe the tools and products they are using; everything must be labeled. Ask them to explain how the products work and how they are supposed to help your feet.

It's okay to ask questions during your service, and your nail technician should be able to answer any questions unless it is outside her scope of practice. At that point, she should say so.

My clients ask a lot of questions, and I love it because it makes me better at my job; it helps me to understand their needs and concerns.

If you don't know what to ask, here are a few questions to get the conversation going. I get asked these questions a lot, and I don't get offended.

How did you get started in this field?
How long have you been doing this?
What kind of additional training do you have in this field?
Do you like what you do?
What kind of products do you use? Why?
Do you work with any doctors?
How do your clients find you?
Do you see a lot of clients with foot issues?
Do you see a lot of clients with health issues?
How long do you plan to do this kind of work?
Do you see any problems with my feet?

These questions should give you a good idea if the person servicing you is a good fit for you.

9

ORTHOTICS

Life is all about balance—mentally, physically, emotionally, and spiritually. Our feet give us telltale signs if we are physically out of balance. We suffer from foot pain, knee pain, hip pain, back pain, and even calluses. These can all be indicators that we are not in balance, that our body is not getting the support it needs.

Generally, when I look at the bottom of a client's feet, if they have calluses on one foot and not the other, they could be favoring one side over the other because they may be suffering from a bad knee or hip. If I see calluses showing up on both feet in the same area, that could be a sign of a lack of support or a foot issue.

At that point, I generally recommend they see a specialist to consider custom orthotics. Custom orthotics are formed to your specific feet to give you the support you need, in the place you need it. I don't generally recommend the ones you find in stores because they may not give you the support you need.

Here are some reasons why custom orthotics can be beneficial:

Prevents injury: Custom orthotics can help prevent injuries by reducing excessive stress and pressure on certain areas of the foot. They provide shock absorption, help maintain proper alignment, and minimize the risk of common injuries like shin splits and Achilles tendinitis.

Reduces foot pain: Custom orthotics are often prescribed to reduce foot pain from conditions like plantar fasciitis, reducing discomfort and promoting pain relief.

Corrects biomechanical issues: Custom orthotics can help with correcting issues like overpronation (excessive inward rolling of the foot) and improving overall foot function.

I am by no means a doctor. However, being someone who has had custom orthotics, I have reaped the benefits of having them and can speak firsthand about the benefits and support they provide.

If you have custom orthotics and you have had them for a while—over a year—it may be time to get them checked to make sure they are still providing the support your body needs.

10

BONUS FOOT CARE TIPS

Here are some tips to keep your feet healthy and clean.

Nail Polish
Nail polish should not be worn over infected toenails (thick, discolored, or brittle).

Gel polish will damage toenails.

Polish should not be worn on toenails for more than three to four weeks.

It is possible for nail polish to crack or lift, causing trapped moisture to get in and cause discoloration and possibly infect a toenail.

Toenails thrive in a healthy environment; nail tincture or nail oil should be used regularly.

Shoes
Never try shoes on in the store without a sock or stocking; fungal toenails or athlete's foot spread easily.

A well-fitting shoe not only supports your feet but also balances your body from your knees and hips to your back.

Soft, comfortable shoes aren't a good fit if they don't provide the support you need.

Just because a shoe feels small, it doesn't always mean you need to go up a size. You may need to try another brand.

Wear the proper shoe for your activity—a running shoe is for runners, a basketball shoe is to play basketball, etc.

If you do not find a shoe that gives you the support you need, try a custom orthotic.

Pedicures

Pedicures should last 24–48 hours after service.

Pedicures or routine foot care should be done every four to six weeks depending on how fast your toenails grow and if you aren't able to cut them safely yourself.

To make your pedicures last longer, you must do daily home care if you are physically able.

Waterless pedicures work with your feet in their natural state to address the actual problem.

Waterless pedicures prevent cross contamination of fungus and bacteria.

Pedicures should be done for self-care and self-health.

Home Care Tools

Tools for home use should only be used by one person. Do not share tools.

Tools for home use should be washed and dried after every use.

Tools for home use should not sit in water for an extended period.

Toenails

Toenails should always be kept short for safety.

Never pick your toenails with your fingernails. You can break and damage both the toenail and fingernail.

When cutting toenails, make sure to finish with a nail file to smooth and even the toenails and their edges.

11

DOCTOR'S CORNER

It is always great to get referrals for my business, but it is a humbling experience when the referral comes from a podiatrist. In my business, I take my work seriously, and the foot care I give to my clients goes beyond just pretty feet. I am nowhere near the level of a doctor, but to know there are doctors out there who trust me enough to send me their patients speaks volumes to me for my work.

Although we have many podiatrists that refer their patients to us, Dr. Baca has by far sent the most and continues to send patients our way.

I wanted this book to be about more than just my words and experiences. I wanted you to hear from a doctor, so when I reached out to Dr. Baca, he was willing to share some, simple but important tips from a podiatrist's perspective on what patients can do to help podiatrists help them.

Dr. Baca understands the dynamics of what I do at FreshSteps Medical Foot and Nail Spa® to help his patients with their foot care and how our connection truly benefits the patient.

Who is Dr. Baca?
John Baca, DPM, FACFAS, FFPM RCPS(Glasg), offers both conservative and surgical care for foot and ankle injuries. He founded Total Foot and Ankle to provide quality podiatry care to patients of all ages. Dr. Baca completed his surgical residency at the Western Pennsylvania Hospital in Pittsburgh, PA. As part of his training, he dedicated time to correcting pediatric limb deformities for underprivileged children in San Salvador, El Salvador. Dr. Baca is currently the medical director of the Department of Podiatry at Medical City Plano Hospital. He has also worked on numerous innovative research projects, including weight-bearing protocols for many procedures.

> Top Plano Podiatrist 2021 by *Dallas Magazine*
>
> Noted Plano podiatrist, Dr. John Baca, is the founder of Total Foot and Ankle in Plano, TX. His state-of-the-art podiatry clinic provides specialized care of the foot and ankle.

Dr. Baca utilizes the latest advancements in treatment including minimally invasive techniques and complex surgical care.

Whether you are a weekend warrior, or a professional athlete, Dr. Baca and his medical staff have the expertise to treat your injury.

We believe in finding treatment solutions that get our patients back to living a pain-free lifestyle. We are accepting new patients!

Below, I have listed five things Dr. Baca shared that you should know.

1) Healthy feet habits
-Wash your feet regularly, even between the toes. This is often a forgotten step while bathing but can be vital in preventing infection.

-Check your feet visually. If it's difficult to see the bottom of your feet or heels, ask a partner for help or place a mirror on the floor to help.

-Avoid walking for long periods without shoes or sandals, especially outdoors. This will prevent puncture wounds or sores.

2) Seek professional help
-If you are unable to bear weight on the lower extremity because of pain or deformity for any reason

-For evaluation of even small wounds or cuts that don't heal within a few days

-Worsening skin discoloration or changes in skin temperature over a short period of time

3) Top illnesses that affect foot health
-Diabetes mellitus

-Peripheral neuropathy

-Peripheral vascular disease

4) Why is proper shoe fit important?
-Proper shoe fit can prevent pain, prevent skin wounds and blisters or nail injuries, and falls during sports activities.

5) Three things a physician needs to know
-How long has the problem been present? Long-term issues can become more complex and difficult to treat.

-Has the problem changed over time? Deformity that is progressive or pain that changes with activity is often concerning.

-What makes the pain better? Has over-the-counter medication, rest, or changes in shoe gear helped alleviate the discomfort?

CONCLUSION

I sincerely hope that the information in this book serves you well and that you can use this information and share it with others to spread awareness about the basic need of maintaining healthy feet.

If you are in the Dallas Fort Worth, Texas area and need help with foot care, we hope you will come visit FreshSteps Medical Foot and Nail Spa® LLC in McKinney, Texas. If you are too far to visit, we do have an online store with our professional products for sale—the same products we use in our salon. You are more than welcome to call and ask questions.

Currently, we only have one location with two highly skilled and advanced trained technicians, but you can follow and subscribe to our YouTube Channel for more tips and the most up-to-date information about our services and any new locations.

Check the resource page for Dr. Baca's information and location and the FreshSteps FootCare information.

RESOURCES

FreshSteps Medical Foot and Nail Spa®
6633 Eldarodo Pkwy, Suite 410
McKinney, Texas 75070
469-850-1520
Email: Freshstepsmedispa@gmail.com
www.freshstepsmediaspa.com
By appointment only
YouTube: FreshSteps Medical Foot and Nail Spa

Purchase Products
FreshSteps FootCare
www.freshstepsfootcare.com
YouTube: FreshSteps FootCare

John Baca, DPM, FACFAS, FFPM RCPS(Glasg)
www.totalfootandankletx.com
6300 Parker Rd, Ste 425
Plano, Texas 75093
(972) 942-8080

Made in the USA
Columbia, SC
09 July 2024